Low Carb

For Rapid Weight Loss, Regaining Confidence and Healing Your Body With Top Delicious & Simple Low Carb Meal Plan Recipes

Richard Leonard

Published by Jason Thawne Publishing House

Low Carb: For Rapid Weight Loss, Regaining Confidence and Healing Your Body With Top Delicious & Simple Low Carb Meal Plan Recipes

ISBN 978-1-989749-45-6

monetary loss due to the information herein, either directly or indirectly.

Respective authors own all copyrights not held by the publisher.

The information herein is offered for just informational purposes solely, and is universal as so. The presentation of the information is without contract or any type of guarantee assurance.

The trademarks that are used are without any consent, and also the publication of the trademark is without permission or backing by the trademark owner. All trademarks and brands within this book are for clarifying purposes only and are the owned by the owners themselves, not affiliated with this document.

TABLE OF CONTENTS

Part 1

Introduction

Low carb diet is not new because it is used in the medical community for a variety of reasons. This diet is linked to numerous benefits, such as quick weight loss, control of blood sugar and insulin, trim down your hunger, and reduce the risk of heart diseases and various types of cancers. A low-carb diet is really effective to fight with stubborn fat because it helps you to reduce weight by restricting the amount and type of carbohydrates. This diet focuses on the consumption of healthy fats and protein. Aside from weight loss, a low carb diet is helpful to avoid various health conditions, such as hypertension, cardiovascular disease, and diabetes.

In a short period of time, you can notice the positive effects of this diet on your sugar level and blood cholesterol. Low carb diet decreases the insulin levels in your blood. Insulin is a hormone that regulates fat storage and production of blood sugar. It encourages your body to use glucose as an energy source rather than fat that is stored in your body. Low insulin levels allow your body to burn more fat and use it as a fuel source. Low carb diet strictly reduces all sources of glucose to force the body to burn stored fat. A traditional low card diet focuses on healthy fat, protein and fiber. There is an inverse relationship between carbohydrate and fats in your diet.

Some people increase protein intake in their diet, but normally people like to eat more sugar and carbs along with unhealthy fats. This can be the root cause of various health problems because your body needs healthy fats to control mood, improve brain function and regulate hormones. High-carb or sugary meals can increase your awkward feelings and you will feel grumpy, irritable and tired. Sugar has addictive effects on your brain to increase anxiety, cravings and fatigue. Low carb diet encourages you to reduce consumption of sugar and unhealthy fat in your diet. You can get the advantage of healthy replacements, such as olive oil and coconut oils. These oils act as precursors and antioxidants to support neurotransmitters and molecules of the brain that control mood, memory, energy, and learning.

The human brain is made up of essential fatty acids; therefore, it always requires a constant stream of fats in your diet. Keep it in mind that a strong metabolic process of high-sugar diet may result in the deficiency of omega-3 fatty acids and affect cognitive abilities of your brain. Insulin action and heavy glucose in your body can control the signals of your brain. Low carb diet encourages you to control the consumption of sugar and reduce the chances of a cerebral problem. Carbohydrate diet is really effective to reduce the particular amount of metabolic and cardiovascular risk factors. People with low-carbohydrate diet may experience a greater boost in lipoprotein cholesterol and reduce triglycerides.

HDL (High-Density Lipoprotein) is known as a good cholesterol. LDL and HDL are known as lipoproteins and these are responsible for carrying cholesterol in your blood. LDL carries cholesterol from the liver to the body and HDL carries cholesterol to your liver, away from your body. This cholesterol is recycled or excreted from your body. A Higher level of HDL can reduce the risk of heart diseases. It will be good to follow a low-carb diet and eat food with low fat to increase HDL.

When you consume carbs, these are broken down into sugars or glucose in your digestive tract. They will enter in the digestive tract and increase the blood sugar levels. High blood sugar is not good for your body and the body responds to the insulin that is a hormone. Insulin tells the cells to burn and store glucose to bring it to a normal level. The body of healthy people can quickly respond to insulin to reduce the blood sugar to avoid any harm. A ketogenic diet will help your body respond to insulin and get rid of type 2 disease. A ketogenic diet will keep your body healthy and you can avoid high blood pressure and type II diabetes.

Metabolic Syndrome

The low carb diet is good for the treatment of metabolic syndromes that are associated with the risk of heart diseases and diabetes. There are a few symptoms of metabolic syndrome:

- High blood pressure
- High triglycerides
- Abdominal obesity
- High blood sugar
- Low HDL levels

These symptoms indicate metabolic syndrome and you can follow the Ketogenic diet to avoid these problems. You can improve the health of your brain with the help of this diet.

Possible Risks of Low Carb Diet

With the drastic reduction of carbs, you may experience a number of temporary health effects, such as a headache, bad breath, fatigue, weakness, and constipation. Long-term use of low-carb diet may result in the deficiency of essential mineral and vitamin. It can increase the risk of various chronic diseases. The carbohydrate reduction should be limited to almost 20 grams a day; otherwise, you may experience ketosis. It is a situation in which there is not glucose in your body for energy, and your body is forced to use stored fat. If you want to follow a low-carb diet, then you can include soups, lasagna, frittatas, stuffed vegetables and chicken sausages in your diet.

Chapter 1 – Benefits of Low Carb Recipes

You know that the health benefits of low carb diet are unlimited because besides weight loss, you can enjoy a constant improvement in blood pressure, blood glucose, and blood lipids. Low carb diet is really effective and successful as compared to traditional diets. Traditional diets may advise you to follow a strict diet that may lead to starvation for a longer period of time. If you are following a low carb diet, you can enjoy your favorite meals because recipes are available with special instructions to make your meals healthy and safe for you. This diet enables you to eat 4 to 5 times in a day and these recipes are given for your assistance. There are a few benefits of low carb recipes that will help you to understand their importance:

Reduce Hunger

Foods like butter, coconut oil, nuts, bacon and avocado are allowed for all low carb dieters. These food items are good for your health, but you have to focus on their quantity. Low carb recipes and diet plan prove helpful for you to manage a headache and the bad reaction of your body. Everyone responds differently on the reduction of carbohydrate in their diet. These recipes and plans are designed in a way to help your body to adjust to this diet. With the passage of time, it will be easy for you to deal with food impulses. These recipes will adjust your appetite and you may feel satisfied with smaller portions of food.

Lots of Low Carb Vegetables can be Consumed

The vegetable is an excellent source of carbohydrates. You can also get fiber, minerals, vitamins and other nutrients by consuming these vegetables. You will get long-lasting energy by consuming these vegetables. You should consume vegetables with low-carbohydrate, such as spinach, celery, mushrooms, and tomatoes. These fruits have 4 grams of carbohydrates in each serving. Starchy vegetables are not good for you because these have a higher amount of carbohydrates. Potatoes, corn, peas, and beans are some starchy vegetables with 12 to 37 grams of carbohydrates in each serving. One serving is equal to a ½ cup and you should be very careful while enjoying these vegetables.

Low Carb Fruits with Fiber

The fruits offer fiber, vitamins and minerals as per the needs of your body. Fruits usually have a higher amount of carbohydrates as compared to vegetables; therefore, you should consume them carefully. The berries like cantaloupe, blackberries, strawberries and honeydew have a lower amount of carbohydrates. You can consume an almost ½ cup of these fruits. Keep it in mind that fruits like banana and mangoes have high carbohydrates as compared to others.

Provide Essential Fiber to Your Body

Fiber is equally important to consider while checking the carbohydrate in fruits. The fiber is a carbohydrate that is difficult to break down by the body. It proves helpful in regular digestion and you can get rid of a number of diseases with the help of fiber rich food. Fiber can slow down the digestion and keeps you full for longer hours; therefore, you should consider fruits with low carbohydrates and high fiber content. The fruits with high fiber are blackberries, raspberries, baby spinach and broccoli. In these food items, there are 4 grams of fiber and 8 grams of carbohydrates in each ½ cup serving.

Increase Your Energy

A low-calorie diet can make your body restless and lack energy after a few minutes. Low carb diets will not affect the energy of your body because you can try these delicious recipes to increase the energy of your body. You can notice a significant increase in your stamina and boost in your performance.

Stable Moods

With the help of low carb recipes, your moods will always remain stable. There is no need to worry about transitory emotions and mood swings. You will feel more stable and confident due to healthy food items and a balanced diet.

Forget about Pain and Aches

Ingredients of low carb recipes will gradually reduce inflammation in your body. After a short period of time, you will not worry about joint and muscle pains. Reduction in headaches and heartburn is really common.

Get Rid of Medications

Low car recipes are based on fresh fruits and vegetables that can gradually reduce bad cholesterol in your body, normalize blood sugar and blood pressure and inflammation. As a result, there is no need to spend money on medications. These will also reduce your regular visits to doctors.

Chapter 2 – Foods to Eat and Avoid

During Low Carb Diet

The low-carb diet typically focuses on proteins, such as fish, eggs, meat and non-starchy vegetables. A low-carb diet will help you to reduce the consumption of grains, fruits, bread, sweet items, pasta, and starchy vegetables. You are allowed to take a limited quantity of particular fruits, vegetables, and grains.

While following a low-carb diet, your regular consumption of the carbohydrates will be limited between 60 and 130 grams. By taking this particular quantity of carbohydrates, you will consume 240 to 520 calories. You need to completely restrict the consumption of carbs during the initial stages of the diet and gradually increase the carbohydrates in your diet up to a restricted number. The dietary guidelines of America explain you should consume 900 to 1,300 calories in a day with 225 to 325 grams carbohydrates.

Good Food Items

There are a few food items that are good for your low carb diet. These food items are given to their carb content:

Eggs (Zero Carb)

Eggs are really healthy and notorious food loaded with lots of nutrients that are important for your brain and eyes.

Meats (Almost Zero Carb)

Almost all kinds of meats are close to zero carbs, but be careful about liver, which has almost 5 percent carbs.

Beef (Zero)

It is loaded with B12 and iron; therefore, you can include it in your diet, such as hamburger, steak and ground beef.

Lamb (Zero)

Lamb is good for your health because it offers B12 and iron contents. You can select grass-fed lamb because it is high in fatty acids called CLA (conjugated linoleic acid).

Chicken (Zero)

Chicken is a popular meat all over the world and it has lots of benefits and an excellent source of protein. You can include thighs and wings of chicken in your diet.

Fish and Seafood (Zero)

Fish is really healthy for you because fish meat is high in omega-3 fatty acids, B12, and iodine. Salmon has iodine, B12, and vitamin D3. You can include sardines and trout in your diet. Shellfish has 4 to 5 percent carbs in each 100 grams.

Vegetables

Various vegetables are low in carb, such as cruciferous and leafy green vegetable are low in carb and have a good amount of fiber. Some root vegetables (starchy) like sweet potatoes and potatoes are high in carbs. There are a few vegetables that are safe for your low carb diet:

• Broccoli contains 7 percent carbohydrates and you can include this tasty vegetable in your diet. This vegetable is loaded with vitamin K, C, and fiber.

- Tomatoes are known as berries and fruits, but these are eaten as vegetables to enhance the flavor of your food. 100 grams tomatoes have 4 percent starch and these are loaded with potassium and vitamin C.

- Almost 100 grams onion has 9 percent carbohydrates and these can add amazing flavor to your low card recipes. These are loaded with antioxidants, fiber, and anti-inflammatory compounds.

- Brussels sprouts can be added to your diet because 100-gram sprouts have 7 percent carbohydrates. These will supply vitamin K and C in your body.

- Cauliflower is a versatile vegetable with lots of vitamin C, K, and folate. It has 5 percent carbohydrates in 100 grams.

- Kale is loaded with carotene antioxidants, vitamin C, and K. It can be a good choice for health conscious people because 100-gram kale has 10 percent carbohydrates.

- 100 grams eggplants have 6 percent carbohydrates and high in fiber.

- 100 grams cucumber has 4 percent carbohydrates, water, and a small quantity of vitamin K.

- Bell peppers are famous for their high content of fiber, carotene antioxidants, and vitamin C. Only 100 grams of bell peppers have 6 grams carbohydrates.

- Asparagus has 2 percent carbohydrates and it is high in fiber, vitamin K, carotene antioxidants and vitamin C. Asparagus is high in protein as compared to various other vegetables.

- 100 grams green beans have 7 percent carbohydrates, and a good amount of protein, fiber, vitamin K, vitamin C, potassium, and magnesium.

- Mushrooms have 3 percent carbohydrates and a decent amount of B-vitamins and potassium.

Various other Low-carb Vegetables

- Spinach
- Celery
- Zucchini
- Cabbage

- Swiss chard

Other than starchy root veggies, you are allowed to enjoy every vegetable because almost all vegetables are low in carbs. You can include lots of vegetables in your diet.

Fruits and Berries

Most fruits are high in carbohydrate contents as compared to vegetables; therefore, you have to be very careful, while selecting fruits. You should restrict your fruit intake to almost 1 to 2 pieces in each day. Some fruits like avocados and olives, along with low-sugar berries, such as strawberries are excellent for you. There are a few good choices for low carb diet:

- Only 100 grams avocado offers 8.5 percent carbohydrates. It is loaded with fiber, potassium, and healthy fat.

- Olives offer 6 percent carbohydrates and high content of copper, iron and vitamin E.

- In 100 grams strawberries, you can get 8 percent carbohydrates because this nutrient-dense food is really delicious to eat. They have vitamins C, antioxidants, and manganese.

•   Grapefruits are citrus fruits with 11 percent carbohydrates. They are high in carotene antioxidants and vitamin C.

•   Apricots have 11 percent carbohydrates and it contains plenty of potassium and vitamin C.

•   Other delicious low-carb fruits are Kiwi, lemons, oranges, raspberries and mulberries.

Seeds and Nuts

These are really famous for including in low-carb diet and they are high in fiber, protein and fat with various micronutrients. You can enjoy nuts as snacks and include flaxseed and coconut flour meals in your diet.

•   22 percent carbohydrates are found in 100 grams almonds. These are loaded with vitamin E, fiber, mineral, and magnesium. These are good to promote weight loss without increasing your calorie count.

- Walnuts contain 14 percent carbohydrates and these are rich in omega-3 fatty acid and other nutrients.

- Peanuts are legumes and these are prepared to consume as nuts. These are high in fiber, vitamin E, magnesium, and vitamins. 100 grams peanuts have 16 percent carbohydrates.

- Chia seeds will be a good addition to your diet because these are loaded with 44 percent carbohydrates, high fiber, and dietary fiber. Keep it in your mind that 86 percent carbs in the chia seeds are basically fiber; therefore, digestible carbs are really low.

- Moreover, cashews, hazelnuts, coconuts, macadamia nuts, pistachios, pumpkin seeds, flax seeds and sunflower seeds are also low in carb content.

- Dairy

- If you can tolerate dairy, you can get the advantage of full-fat dairy products because these are excellent in low-carbohydrate diet without added sugar:

• Cheese is a low-carbohydrate food that can be enjoyed raw, or included in different delicious recipes. It goes well with meat and burger. 100 grams cheese has 1.3 grams carbohydrates.

• Heavy cream has 3 percent carbohydrate and a small amount of protein. It is packed with dairy fiber and perfect to enjoy with low-carb desserts.

• Almost 100 grams full-fat yogurt is loaded with probiotic bacteria and 5 percent carbohydrates. Greek yogurt has 4 percent carbohydrates and a good amount of protein.

Oils and Fats

There are various healthy oils and fats that are acceptable to include in your low-carb diet and other weight loss diets. There are a few healthy choices for your assistance:

• Butter has zero carbohydrates and high saturated-fat content. Make sure to use grass-fed butter because it has various essential nutrients.

• Olive Oil (extra virgin) has zero carbohydrates; therefore, it has healthy fat and loaded with powerful anti-inflammatory compounds and antioxidants. It is good for your cardiovascular health.

• Coconut oil can be a good addition to your diet because it can reduce your appetite and help you to reduce belly fat. It has zero carbohydrates and good to increase your metabolism.

• Lard, avocado oil, and tallow will be a good addition to your diet.

Low Carb Beverages

Make sure to avoid fruit juices because these are high in carbs and sugar. Some sugar-free and low carb beverages are as follows:

• Water should be an important part of your diet because it will be you to reduce weight and increase your metabolism. Water is free from carbohydrates and calories.

• Coffee is really healthy with zero carbs and help you to deal with type 2 diabetes, Alzheimer and Parkinson's disease. Make sure to avoid sugar, full-fat cream and heavy cream in coffee.

•	Tea has no carbohydrates and green tea can boost metabolism and fat burning speed. Avoid extra sugar and milk in tea.

•	Carbonated water and club soda are acceptable because there is zero sugar and carbohydrates.

•	Dark chocolate is the perfect treat for low carb diet because cocoa content can improve your brain function and reduce blood sugar. Dark chocolates have many health benefits and 100 grams chocolate has 46 grams carbohydrates. Dark chocolate also has 25 percent fiber of your body.

Condiments, Herbs, and Spices

There are numerous varieties of delicious herbs, condiments, and spices. You can enjoy them without fear because these are low in carbohydrates and add flavor to your meals.

Chapter 3 – Low Carb Recipes for Breakfast

To make your breakfast healthy and delicious, there are a few low carb recipes for you. These are simple and healthy:

Recipe 01: Steak and Eggs with Tomatoes

- 1 teaspoon olive oil

- 1 pound steak

- Salt and black pepper

- 4 medium tomatoes, sliced into halves

- 4 eggs

- 1 tablespoon oregano (fresh and chopped)

DIRECTIONS:

Take a large pan and keep it on a medium heat with 1 dollop of oil. Sprinkle salt and pepper on the steaks. Let them cook for 4 to 5 minutes and turn the sides after that time. Remove the cover and leave the slices in the pan for almost 5 minutes.

Place pieces of tomatoes in the pan and cook them for 2 to 3 minutes to get a brown color.

Now, once again pour the 1 teaspoon of oil on the nonstick skillet on the medium heat. Break the eggs in the nonstick skillet and cover it to cook for almost 2 to 4 minutes. Slightly turn the sunny side of the eggs and sprinkle oregano on the eggs and tomatoes. Add salt and pepper as well to serve them with yummy steaks.

Nutritional Information Per Serving:

305 total calories, 17 g fat, 251 mg cholesterol, 427 mg sodium, 32 g protein, 7 g carbohydrate, 4 g sugar, 2 g fiber, 3 mg iron and 65 mg calcium.

Recipe 02: Eggs with Tomatoes

- 1 teaspoon olive oil

- 1 pound steak

- Salt and black pepper

- 4 medium tomatoes, sliced into halves

- 4 eggs

- 1 tablespoon oregano (fresh and chopped)

DIRECTIONS:

Take a large pan and keep it on a medium heat with 1 dollop of oil. Sprinkle salt and pepper on the steaks. Let them cook for 4 to 5 minutes and turn the sides after that time. Remove the cover and leave the slices in the pan for almost 5 minutes. Place pieces of tomatoes in the pan and cook them for 2 to 3 minutes to get a brown color.

Now, once again pour the 1 teaspoon of oil on the nonstick skillet on the medium heat. Break the eggs in the nonstick skillet and cover it to cook for almost 2 to 4 minutes. Slightly turn the sunny side of the eggs and sprinkle oregano on the eggs and tomatoes. Add salt and pepper as well to serve them with yummy steaks.

Nutritional Information Per Serving:

305 total calories, 17 g fat, 251 mg cholesterol, 427 mg sodium, 32 g protein, 7 g carbohydrate, 4 g sugar, 2 g fiber, 3 mg iron and 65 mg calcium

Recipe 03: Skillet Souffle

- 6 eggs
- ¼ cup chives (chopped and fresh)
- 1 teaspoon salt
- ¼ tsp black pepper
- 1 tablespoon butter without salt
- 4 ounces cheese (Goal Milk)
- 1 5-ounce green salad
- ½ pint grape tomatoes (Sliced in halves)
- 2 tablespoons olive oil
- 1 lemon

DIRECTIONS:

Let the oven heat t 400° F. Take a large bowl and whisk all egg yolks with salt and pepper. Add chives as well in the eggs. Now use an electric mixture to beat the egg whites on a medium speed and mix with the blend of yolk.

Take a large nonstick pan and let the butter melt over it on a medium heat. Coat all the sides of the pan and wait for a few seconds. Add the mixture of eggs on the top of the pan and bake the eggs for almost 10 minutes to get a golden color. Cut the egg into bars and garnish the soufflé with green salad and tomatoes. Sprinkle olive oil and serve with lemon.

Nutritional Information Per Serving

72 calories from fat, 23 g fat, 688 mg Sodium, 16 g Protein, 4 g Carbohydrates, 3 g sugar and 1 g fiber.

Recipe 04: Herbal Eggs

- 1 ½ tablespoons butter without salt
- 8 eggs
- 2 tablespoons milk or water
- Salt
- Ground black pepper
- ½ cup chopped herbs, including parsley and tarragon)
- Take green parts of scallions

DIRECTIONS:

Take a nonstick pan, pour butter and let it heat over a medium flame. In the meantime, take a large bowl and whisk all eggs at one place with milk, salt, and pepper. Pour this mixture into the frying pan and then cook it almost 4 to 5 minutes. Turn it upside down occasionally and sprinkle with herbs and green scallions.

Nutritional Information Per Serving:

183.2 total calories, 13.6-gram fat, 5.38 grams sat fat, 432.64 mg cholesterol, 370.31 mg sodium, 13 mg protein, 1.5 g carbohydrates, 0.23 g fiber, 2.23 mg iron and 69.64 mg calcium.

Recipe 05: Greek Frittata

- Olive oil 3 tablespoons
- 10 whole eggs
- 2 salt
- ½ teaspoon fresh and ground pepper
- 1 5-ounce baby spinach
- 1-pint grape tomatoes (Slices)
- 4 scallions (sliced)
- 8ounces feta, crushed

DIRECTIONS:

Preheat the oven to 350° F and add oil in a casserole. Keep it in the oven for 5 minutes, and during this time, you can whisk eggs, pepper, and salt together. It is time to add tomato, scallions and spinach as well. Gently swirl the feta and take out casserole from the oven. Transfer mixture into casserole and bake it for 25 to 30 minutes to get puffed and golden color eggs.

Nutritional Information:

461 total calories, 65 g fat, 579 mg cholesterol, 1,868 mg sodium, 26 g protein, 8 g carbohydrate, 5 g sugar, and 2 g fiber.

Recipe 06: Creamy Baked Eggs Garnished

with Herbs

- 1 tablespoon soft butter without salt

- 8 tablespoons low fat cream

- 8 whole eggs

- Salt as per taste

- Ground black pepper

- 1 tablespoon fresh parsley and dill (chopped)

- Toast (at the time of serving)

DIRECTIONS:

Preheat your oven to 425° F and take eight ramekins and coat it with cream. Break 2 eggs in the ramekin and sprinkle salt and pepper. In each ramekin, place 2 tablespoons cream. Keep them in the oven for 10 to 12 minutes and sprinkle parsley and dill for additional flavor.

Nutritional Information Per Serving:

271 total calories, 24 g fat, 471 mg cholesterol, 392 mg sodium, 13 g protein, 2 g carbohydrates, 1 g sugar, 0 g fiber, 2 mg iron and 74 mg calcium.

Recipe 07: Low Carb Blender Pan Cake

- 2 cups oats

- 2 cups cottage cheese (low-fat)

- 4 teaspoons baking powder

- 2 cups egg whites

- 2-3 teaspoon sweetener

- 1 teaspoon vanilla

INSTRUCTIONS:

Take 2 cup oats and blend in the blender to make a fine powder. It is time to add 2 cups cottage cheese and egg whites. Add almost 4 teaspoon baking powder and 3 teaspoon sweetener. It will be good to use honey instead of white sugar. You can add vanilla and blend it well. Take a nonstick frying pan and place it on the medium heat. Pour mixture and let it cook by turning its sides. You can make almost 18 to 20 large pancakes.

Recipe 08: Rainbow Vegetable Noodles

- 1 Average Zucchini

- 1 Average Summer Squash

- 1 Carrot

- 1 Thin Sweet Potato

- 4 oz. Onion (Red)

- 6 oz. Bell Peppers (Yellow, orange, and Red)

- 3 Garlic Cloves

- 4 tablespoons butter

- Salt and Pepper As per your taste

DIRECTIONS:

Let the oven heat at 400° and use butter to grease the baking sheets. A spiral slicer will help you to crush the zucchini, carrot, sweet potato and carrot. You will get colorful ribbons to set in a bowl. Combine all vegetables, sprinkle salt and pepper. Mix them well and spread on the baking sheet just like noodles. Bake them for almost 20 minutes and then fold for 10 minutes.

Nutritional Ingredients Per Servings:

48 total calories, 1.5 g protein, 8 g carbs, 1 gram fat.

For healthy lunch options during a low carb diet, there are a few recipes for you to follow:

Recipe 10: Low Carb Cauliflower Salad

- 1 cauliflower (Head)
- 1 lb shrimp (raw)
- 1 tablespoon olive oil
- 2 cucumbers
- 3 tablespoon dill, sliced
- ¼ cup olive oil
- ¼ cup lemon juice
- 2 tablespoons shredded lemon zest
- Salt & Pepper as per taste

Directions:

Completely clean the shrimps, remove the tail and put the raw shrimps on the cookie sheet. Sprinkle 1 tablespoon of olive oil and sprinkle salt and pepper. Heat the oven to 350 degrees and cook the shrimps for almost 10 minutes. There is no need to overcook because the shrimps will be chewy.

Cut the florets of the cauliflower and throw the bottom stalk. Chop them into small pieces and bake the cauliflower in the microwave for almost 5 minutes. You just need to make it soft and you can do it in two batches. Let your shrimp and cauliflower to cool down and chop the cucumber into slices. After cooling down shrimps, you can combine both shrimps and cucumber in a medium bowl. Put some lemon zest and dill with olive oil and lemon juices. Mix it well and then season it with spices.

Nutritional Information per Serving:

214 total calories, 13 g fat, 5 g carbohydrates and 17 g protein.

Recipe 11: Chicken Shawarma with Basil

Lemon

- 1 lbs chicken breast, 3-inch strips
- Olive oil (2 tablespoons)

- Lemon juice (2 tablespoons)
- ¾ teaspoon sea salt
- 3 cloves of garlic (finely chopped)
- 1 teaspoon curry (ground)
- ½ teaspoon cumin (Powder)
- ¼ teaspoon coriander (powder)

Salad

- 6 cups spring greens
- 1 cup cherry tomatoes (sliced)
- 2 handful basil leaves (fresh)
- 1 avocado, chopped

Basil-Lemon Vinaigrette

- 2 handfuls basil leaves
- 1 clove garlic, chopped
- ½ teaspoon sea salt
- 2 tablespoons lemon sap
- 5 tablespoons olive oil

Directions:

Take a bowl and beat olive oil, lemon juice, salt, garlic, cumin powder, coriander to mix them well. Take a large bag with zipping and add chicken strips for marination. Keep it in the refrigerator for almost 20 minutes. You can also marinate it for one night.

If you want to make the meal, you can take a frying pan and keep it on a medium heat. Add a small quantity of olive oil and cook chicken to get a golden brown color. You need to cook it for almost 6 to 8 minutes to make the juices clear.

In a food processor, add basil, salt, lemon juice and garlic and process it. You can also add oil and blend the mixture to combine everything. Greens will help you to make a salad and add some salt and pepper. Add chicken on the tops of greens with basil, tomatoes, and avocado.

Nutrition facts

One serving contains 392 calories, 28 grams of fat, 9 grams of carbs and 27 grams of protein.

Recipe 12: Low Carb Avgolemono (Greek Chicken, Lemon & Egg Soup)

Take a large saucepan and pour chicken broth and shredded chicken to let them simmer. When they come to the boiling point, remove from the heat and keep them aside. Take a medium bowl and beat eggs and lemon juice together to get a frothy mixture. Slowly mix 2 cups of hot stock into the mixture and let them incorporate properly. Be careful, and don't dump the mixture; otherwise, the eggs can be scrambled. Pour this mixture into the saucepan and mix the shredded squash into the soup and reheat it. Let it boil and then sprinkle spices.

Make sure to serve hot and add chopped parsley and cheese.

Nutritional Information:

289 calories, 15g fat, 4g net carbs, and 33g protein

Recipe 14: Spaghetti Squash of Kale and

Mushroom

Crust

- 1 medium crushed spaghetti

- 1/2 tsp parsley
- 1/2 tsp onion
- 1/4 tsp salt

Filling:

- 3 cups chopped mushrooms
- 1 chopped onion
- 5 crushed garlic cloves
- 2 cups kale
- 2 eggs
- 1 cup egg whites
- 1 cup cheese
- 1 cup cottage cheese
- 2 tsp garlic powder
- 1 1/2 tsp dried thyme
- 1/2 tsp salt
- 3/4 tsp black pepper, ground
- Cooking spray

Directions:

Let the oven heat to 400 degrees F and cut the squash in two halves to place on the baking sheet. Use a parchment paper to bake the squash for 30 minutes.

On the other side, take a frying pan, grease it and keep it on a high heat. Sauté mushrooms for 5 minutes to get a golden brown color. Shift the mushrooms in the medium bowl and keep the frying pan again on medium flame after greasing it again. Fry garlic and onion for 2 minutes in the frying pan and add kale, salt, black pepper and basil as well to sauté them. Add these things in a bowl of mushroom and set it aside.

Add garlic, onion, salt, and thyme to add in a medium bowl. Seed the squash with the help of a fork to make the crust. Transfer this to a deep pie dish and keep on a side. Whisk egg, add cheese, kale and garlic powder, basil, salt and pepper to make a perfect blend. Pour this blend into the crust and let the squash absorb the liquid. Bake it at 400 degrees F for 50 minutes. Leave it for 30 minutes after removing from oven and then cut into 8 slices.

Nutritional Information Per Serving:

Calories: 170.1, Fat: 6.4 g, Cholesterol: 61.5 mg, Sodium: 498.4 mg, Total Carbs: 14.5 g, Dietary Fiber: 3.3 g, Protein: 14.0 g

Recipe 15: Buffalo Chicken Wraps with Lettuce

- 2 cooked chicken breasts shred meat
- 2 tablespoons butter
- 1/2 tablespoon olive oil
- 1/2 cup Wing Sauce
- 1/2 tsp. salad leaves
- Ground black pepper
- 1/2 Cup sliced celery
- Cheese crush
- Salad Dressing
- Lettuce heads

Directions:

Take a large skillet to cook your chicken with a ½ cup of water. Shred it and drain all water. Keep the pan on medium heat, add butter and stir it. Add the salad leaves and dressing with some pepper powder. Let the sauce simmer and then remove from the heat. Sprinkle salary leaves and pour the mixture on the leaves of lettuce. Serve it warm.

Recipe 16: Fried Chicken Breast

- Butter
- Chicken Breast
- Seat Salt
- Black ground Pepper
- Garlic Powder
- Curry and vegetables

Directions:

Cut the chicken into small pieces and then add butter in the pan to stir fry the chicken pieces. Add some salt, pepper, garlic powder and curry powder in the frying pan. Wait for the brown color and after getting your desired results, you can serve with salad.

Recipe 17: Tuna Salad without Mayo

- 5-oz tuna
- 1 tablespoon olive oil
- 1 teaspoon mustard

- 1 boiled egg (chopped finely)
- 1/2 celery stalk, minced
- Salt
- Black pepper powder
- 4 romaine leaves of large size
- 1 teaspoon diced parsley

Directions:

Take a tune, mustard, olive oil, boiled eggs, salt and black pepper to mix in one bowl. Keep each piece of tuna on a large leaf and sprinkle basil. If you are looking to consume in the lunch, then prepare in the morning and for the dinner, prepare it at the lunch time. Refrigerate the tune to make it ready to consume. When you need to consume it, you can bake tuna and consume with chopped eggs and celery.

Nutritional Information Per Serving:

352 calories, 20.2 g fat, 3.6 g carbohydrate, 1.7 g fiber, 0.2 g sugars, 39.4 g protein, 739 mg sodium, 244 mg cholesterol

Recipe 18: Pesto Zucchini Delicious

Noodles

- 4 medium zucchini, sliced
- Salt as per taste
- 6 pieces of uncooked bacon
- 1/2 cup onions, sliced
- 2 cups broccoli flowers
- 2-3 basil pesto (teaspoon)
- Fresh cheese, for garnish

DIRECTIONS:

Cut the zucchini and keep it in a bowl and season with salt. Mix the ingredients and let them aside for 15 minutes. Remove additional water and squeeze the zucchini, if required. Cook bacon in a frying pan to make it crispy and keep them on a paper towel to absorb additional heat.

Add green onion and broccoli in the pan while keeping it on a medium heat and let it cook for 3 to 5 minutes. Put zucchini and pesto, stir well and combine all ingredients in one bowl. You can add additional pesto to enhance the taste. You can blaze it for 2 minutes at the time of serving and serve with grated cheese.

To make your low carb dinner special, there are a few delicious recipes that are simply amazing for everyone:

Recipe 19: Spinach Soup

- 25g butter (low-fat)
- Spring onions chopped only 1 bunch
- 120-gram leek, chopped
- 85 g celery (about 2 small sticks), sliced
- 200 g potatoes (1 medium), peel it properly and divide into pieces
- ½ tsp black pepper (freshly ground)
- Make stock (made with two chicken or vegetable stock cubes)
- 2 bags spinach
- 150g half-fat cream

Directions:

Take a large saucepan and let the butter melt, and now add onions, potatoes, celery and leek. Mix them well and put a lid on the pot to let them cook for 10 minutes. Keep stirring them and after 10 minutes, add stock in it. Now you will cook it for another 10 to 15 minutes until the potatoes and other vegetables become soft. In the end, add spinach and let it cook for a few minutes. You can blend the soup in a blender to make a smooth paste and mix the low-fat cream. Reheat the soup before serving it.

Nutritional Information:

192 calories, 6.5g protein, 13.1g carbs, 12.6g fat, 7.2g saturated fat, 5.4g fiber, 4.4g sugar, and 2g salt.

Recipe 20: Delicious Rainbow Soup

- 1 medium onion, chopped

- Celery should be Properly chopped, 2 large stalks

- 4 cloves garlic, crushed

- 1 medium bell pepper (Red)

- 1 cup chopped carrot or pumpkin

- 1 full teaspoon of sweet paprika

- 3 teaspoons turmeric powder

- 1/2 teaspoon cinnamon

- 1 bay leaf

- Hot sauce

- Chopped tomatoes

- A green chard leaf and cut it into strips. (You can also use other green leafy vegetables like spinach or kale).

- Green beans almost 10 oz,

- Salt and pepper,

- 5 cups broth

- 1 tablespoon olive oil

Directions:

Add oil, onion, celery in a large pot and cook it for 5 to 10 minutes to make onion sweet. It is time to put garlic into it and then reduce the heat to medium. Let them cook for a few minutes and then add peppers as well as carrots. Cook for another minute before adding spices.

Now you will add tomato paste and stock to let it cook for almost 15 minutes. Add beans and chard and let the soup boil for 5 minutes to let the beans properly cooked. At this time, you can also add shredded meat.

Nutritional Information:

Servings, 9 cups of 6 grams, carbohydrate and 3 grams of fiber (9 grams total carbohydrate) and 53 calories.

Recipe 21: Carrot Soup with Coriander

Flavor

- 1 tbsp vegetable oil

- 1 onion, sliced

- 1.2 lb vegetable stock (chicken stock can also be used)

- 1 potato, sliced

- 450g carrots chopped after peeling

- 1 tsp ground coriander

- Handful coriander (1/2 packet)

Directions:

Take a large pan and add onion to let them fry for 5 minutes. Add coriander and potato to cook for 1 minute and add the carrots and broth to let them boil. At this point, reduce the heat and cover the pot for 20 minutes to make carrots soft. You can blend it in a blender to make everything smooth. Reheat while serving it.

Nutritional Information:

Calories 115, Protein 3g, Carbs 19g, Fat 4g, Saturates 1g, Fiber 5g, Sugar 12g, Salt 0.46g.

Recipe 22: Chicken Vegetable Soup

- 1 small or 1/2 large onion, cut into pieces
- 2 stalks celery, cut into small pieces
- 1 large carrot, cut into small pieces
- 1 tablespoon olive oil
- 3 cloves garlic, crushed
- 1-quart chicken broth
- 1 cup chicken meat (cooked and chopped)
- 1/3 cup salsa
- 1/8 teaspoon black pepper

- 1/4 cup chopped leafy herbs like parsley, celery leaves, or oregano.

- Vegetables of your choice

Directions:

Stir fry the onion and vegetable of your choice in a soup pot and then add garlic and fry for one minute. It is time to add broth, vegetables, and salt, but doesn't add green vegetables at the start. The green vegetables should be added at the end to avoid overcooking. Let the stock boil and cook on a medium heat to properly cook all vegetables. You may need more water to cook vegetables and then add low-fat butter, spices, and herbs and cook for one minute. Serve hot for better taste.

Nutritional Information:

5 grams of serving contains 5 grams carbohydrate and 1.5 grams of fiber, 11 grams of protein, and 92 calories.

Recipe 23: Special Italian Fish Soup

- 8 ounces fresh sea bass fillets

- 6 ounces deveined shrimp

- 1/3 cup sliced onion

- 2 stalks sliced celery

- 1/2 teaspoon minced garlic

- 2 teaspoons olive oil

- 1 cup chicken broth (low salt)

- 1 14 diced tomatoes, without salt

- 1 teaspoon dried oregano, chopped

- 1/4 teaspoon salt

- 1/8 teaspoon freshly ground pepper

- 1 tablespoon fresh parsley

Directions:

Defrost fish and shrimp and rinse properly. Let them dry on a white paper town and then cut into pieces. The shrimp should be cut in lengthwise halves. You need to cook onion, garlic and celery in hot oil in a large saucepan and add broth. Let the mixture boil for 5 minutes and mix tomato sauce, oregano, and spices. Let them boil again and cover the pot for 5 minutes.

Carefully mix fish and shrimp and let them boil on a low heat for 5 minutes to let the fish flake easily and shrimp opaque. Garnish parsley before serving hot.

Nutritional Information in Each Serving:

165 gram each serving, Fat 4 g, carb 12 g, 2 g fiber, 19 mg sodium

Recipe 24: Bacon-Cheddar Cauliflower

Broth

- 8 slices bacon, sliced
- 1/2 small chopped onion
- 1 chopped celery stalk
- 2 garlic cloves, crushed
- Salt
- Black Pepper
- 4 cups chopped cauliflower
- 2 Tablespoons gluten-free flour
- 2 cups chicken chowder
- 2 cups milk
- Hot sauce as per needs
- 2-1/2 cups cheddar cheese
- 2 onions, chopped and green

Directions:

Mix chicken and flour together in a small bowl, and keep it on a side. Now cook the bacon in a large pot on a medium heat. Transfer the bacon on towel paper with spoon having slots and keep this plate aside. You can cook celery, chopped onion, garlic and vegetable for 4 to 5 minutes. Sprinkle salt and pepper to cook them well.

Pour water in the pot, add water and let it cook for 5 to 7 minutes. Pour leftover chicken broth and milk in the pot and let it simmer. Slowly mix the broth and chicken and flour, and let it cook again for 3 to 4 minutes. Turn off the flame and mix 2 cups of cheese and mix well to get a smooth texture. Adjust the salt and pepper as per your taste and add hot sauce to enhance its flavor. Use grated cheese while serving it with onion and bacon.

Nutritional Information Per Serving:

Serves 8, 265 calories, 7 grams of carbs, and 15 grams of protein per serving

Recipe 25: Burger with Mushrooms

- Portabella Burgers
- 4 mushroom caps
- 3 ½ tablespoons vinegar
- 2 tablespoons olive oil
- 2 sliced tomatoes
- 2 sliced halloumi
- Sea salt
- Black Pepper
- 1 handful of sage leaves

Directions:

Let the grill heat over 450 degrees and in the meantime, wash mushroom caps. Take a shallow bowl and mix olive oil and vinegar. Mix the mushrooms in the blend and keep the mushroom on the grill for almost 5 minutes. Flip it 2 to 3 times and add halloumi for 2 minutes to the grill. Cook it on high heat and pour cheese over it. Season it with salt and pepper. Assemble the burger with tomato, mushroom, cheese and basil leaves. Serve hot with additional sauce.

Recipe 26: Vegetable Beef Soup with

Pepper Corn

- 2 pounds Beef for stew

- 32 oz beef chowder

- 15 oz sliced tomatoes

- 1 Bay leaf

- 5 peppercorns

- 1 teaspoon sodium

- ¼ teaspoon fresh thyme leaves

- ¼ teaspoon marjoram herb

- 1 medium diced onion

- 1 large carrot

- ½ lb. green beans, chopped

- 1 stick of celery

Directions:

Prepare stew meat and cut into pieces. Take a large pot and heat olive oil to cook the beef. Make sure to cook it until it becomes brown and add 32 oz. of broth into it. Add spices, marjoram, and peppercorns and cover the pot to let it simmer to tender the beef. It may take 2 to 3 hours. Cut all vegetables into small pieces and add in thebroth with tomatoes to cook for 60 to 90 minutes. Make sure to cover the pot with a lid and check the vegetables before removing it from heat.

Chapter 6 – Low Carb Dessert Recipes

If you want to satisfy your sweet tooth, you can try these low carb dessert recipes because these are really great for everyone:

Recipe 27: Pecan Coconut Chocolate Chip

- 2 1/2 cups gluten-free flour

- 1 teaspoon baking soda

- 1 cup butter (plain and flavored)

- 1/2 teaspoon salt

- Sweet cream (2 tablespoons)

- 1/2 cup brown sugar

- 2 eggs

- 2 teaspoon coconut + vanilla extract

- 1 1/2 cups coconut flakes

- 1 cup crushed pecans

- 3/4 cup chocolate chips (black and white)

Directions:

Set the temperature of an oven to 350 degrees F, and let it heat. Prepare a baking sheet with parchment paper and keep it aside. Take a bowl and mix butter and brown sugar. In another bowl, you will prepare the mixture of salt, flour and baking soda. Beat eggs and mix coconut extracts and vanilla. Mix all the ingredients in one bowl and blend the mixture well. Use a tablespoon to evenly distribute the mixture on the baking sheet with a distance of almost one inch. Place the baking sheet in oven for almost 13 to 15 minutes. Remove from the oven after baking them and let them cool down slightly before sprinkling chocolate.

Nutrition Information for Each Cookie:

Calories 186, Fat, 11.3, Cholesterol 18, Sodium 103, Sugars 12.4, Dietary Fiber 1, Protein 2.1, Potassium 54, Total carbohydrates 20.1

Recipe 28: Red Velvet Low Carb Cookies

- 15oz Kidney Beans

- 1/2 cup roasted Beet pulp

- 1/4 cup Almond Milk

- 2 tsp coconut flakes

- 2 tsp butter flavor

- 1 tsp Stevia flakes

- 1/4 tsp Salt

- ¾ cup Erythritol 53g

- 2/3 cup Cocoa Powder without sugar

- ¼ cup white flour

- 2 tsp Baking Powder

- 1 tsp White Vinegar

Directions:

In a food processor, process kidney beans, almond milk, and extracts to get a smooth blend. Add erythritol and puree as well to get a smooth blend. Set the temperature of an oven to 350 degrees F, and let it heat. Prepare a baking sheet with parchment paper and keep it aside. Mix cocoa powder, flour and bean batter in a bowl to make the batter. Add vinegar to whisk everything to get a smooth texture. Use a tablespoon to evenly distribute the mixture on the baking sheet with a distance of almost one inch. Place the baking sheet in oven for almost 13 to 15 minutes. Remove from the oven after baking them and let them cool down slightly before sprinkling chocolate.

Nutrition Information for Each Cookie:

Total calories 250, Fat 12 g, Sodium 270mg, Sugars 20 g, Total Carbohydrate 25 g, Protein 3 g

Recipe 29: Sugar-Free Cookies

- 1/2 cup butter without salt
- 1 cup Granulated sweetener
- 1 tablespoon vanilla
- 1/4 cup egg alternative
- 1/4 cup water

- 3/4 teaspoon vinegar

- 1/4 teaspoon salt

- 1 1/2 cups flour (all purpose)

- 1 1/2 cups flour for cake

- 1 teaspoon powder for baking

Directions:

Set the temperature of an oven to 350 degrees F, and let it heat. Prepare a baking sheet with parchment paper and keep it aside. Prepare the dough with the help of four, butter, vinegar, water, and all other ingredients. You can use an electric mixer to blend properly. Divide the dough equally, and cut it with a cookie cutter to place on the baking sheet with a distance of almost one inch. Place the baking sheet in oven for almost 10 to 12 minutes. Remove from the oven after baking them and let them cool down slightly before sprinkling chocolate.

Nutrition Information for Each Cookie:

Calories 60, Fat 3 g, Sodium 30 mg, Total Carbs 7g, Sugars 1 g and Protein 1 g

Recipe 30: Oatmeal Cookies

- 1 1/2 cups oats (old fashioned)

- 1/2 cup flour (all purpose)

- 1/2 cup gluten free flour

- 2 teaspoon cinnamon powder

- 1/2 teaspoon baking soda

- 1/4 teaspoon salt

- 1/3 cup vegetable butter

- 1/2 cup brown sugar

- 1 whole egg

- 1/4 cup raisins

- 1 teaspoon vanilla flakes

Directions:

Set the temperature of an oven to 350 degrees F, and let it heat. Prepare a baking sheet with parchment paper and keep it aside. Mix butter and sugar in a blender. Take another bowl to mix the rest of the ingredients one by one. Make a dough by mixing the contents of both the bowls. Use a tablespoon to evenly distribute the mixture on the baking sheet with a distance of almost one inch. Place the baking sheet in oven for almost 13 to 15 minutes. Remove from the oven after baking them and let them cool down slightly before sprinkling chocolate.

Nutrition Information for Each Cookie:

Calories 98 g, Total Fat 3 g, Total Carbohydrates 17 g, Sugars 8 g, Dietary Fiber 1 g, and Protein 2 g.

Recipe 31: Gingerbread Cookies

- 1/4 cup soft butter
- 1/4 cup vegetable oil spread
- 1/2 cup sugar (brown)
- 2 teaspoons ginger (powder)
- 1 teaspoon baking soda
- 1 teaspoon cinnamon (powder)
- 1/4 teaspoon cloves (powder)
- 1/4 teaspoon salt
- 1/4 cup molasses (flavored)
- 1 egg
- 2 cups flour (all-purpose)
- 3/4 cup gluten-free flour

Directions:

Set the temperature of an oven to 350 degrees F, and let it heat. Prepare a baking sheet with parchment paper and keep it aside. Take a large bowl and mix butter, vegetable oil spread and beat for almost 30 seconds with an electric mixer. It is time to add ginger, baking soda, salt, cloves, sugar and cinnamon to mix them well. It is time to add flours and mingle to make a dough. Split the dough in half and keep in the refrigerator for almost 2 to 3 hours.

Roll the dough and use a gingerbread cookie cutter to cut out the shapes. Place them on a baking sheet and keep it in the oven for almost 5 to 7 minutes. Remove from the oven after baking them and let them cool down slightly before sprinkling chocolate.

Nutrition Information for Each Cookie:

Calories 73, Fat 2 g, Sodium, 73 mg, Carbohydrates 12 g and Protein 1 gram.

Chapter 7 – Low Carb Sauces, Seasoning, and Condiments

There are some seasoning, spices, sauces and condiments that can enhance the flavors of your food:

Italian Sausage Seasoning

- Italian seasoning: 2 teaspoons
- Parsley: 2 teaspoons
- Minced Garlic: 1 tablespoon
- Minced Onions: 1 teaspoon
- Black pepper: 1 1/2 teaspoons
- Red pepper flakes: 1 teaspoon
- Fennel: 1/2 teaspoon
- Salt: 2 teaspoons
- Paprika: 1/2 teaspoon
- Ground beef: 2 pounds

Directions:

Take a small bowl and prepare a mixture of all the seasonings. You can secure this mixture in a glass jar and add in 2 pounds ground beef or any other meat.

Chili Seasoning Mix

•   Chili powder: 1 teaspoon or more as per your taste

•   Garlic powder: 1 teaspoon

•   Red pepper (crushed flakes): 1/2 teaspoon

•   Paprika: 2 teaspoons

•   Ground cumin: 1 1/2 teaspoons

•   Dried oregano: 1/2 teaspoon

•   Black pepper: 1/2 teaspoon

•   Ground cloves: 1 pinch

•   Sea salt: 1/2 teaspoon

•   Ground cinnamon: 1 pinch

•   Onion powder: 1 teaspoon or you can crush fried and dried onion and use 2 teaspoons

Directions:

Mix all the ingredients in a bowl and select an airtight container to store it in a cool place.

Fish Spice Mix

- Crushed rosemary (Dried): 1 tablespoon

- Black pepper powder: 2 teaspoons

- Dried basil: 1 tablespoon

- Celery salt: 1 teaspoon

- Dried parsley: 1 tablespoon

- Sea salt: 2 teaspoons

- Dry sage powder: 2 teaspoons

- Thyme leaves (dried): 2 teaspoons

- Oregano leaves (dried): 1 teaspoon

- Marjoram leaves (dried): 2 teaspoons

- Garlic powder: 1 teaspoon

Directions:

You can combine thyme, black pepper, rosemary, celery salt, parsley, basil, oregano, marjoram, sea salt, garlic powder and sage in a bowl to make an equal blend. You have to store this blend in an airtight container.

Recipe: Mint Sauce

- 1/8 cup mint leaves, fresh

- ¼ cup pure butter

- 2 packs Splenda

Directions:

Blend all ingredients on low heat and serve with chicken or lamb. The entire recipe has 2 grams net carbs.

Recipe: White Sauce

- Butter: 2 Tablespoon

- Heavy Cream: 1/2 cup

- Full-Fat Soy (Flour): 2 Tablespoon

- Cold Water: 1/2 cup

- Egg yolks: 2 large

- Salt as per taste

- One pinch White Pepper

Directions:

Start your work by melting butter in a saucepan over low heat. With the help of wire whisk, you can mix soy flour and cook it for a few minutes to make a smooth blend. Now, combine water and cream, slowly add the butter and flour mixture in this blend. Use wire to mix and add pepper and salt as per taste. Heat it to scald it and beat eggs in yolks. You shouldn't let this blend boil. It will make almost one cup sauce and this whole recipe has 8 grams carbohydrates.

Chapter 8 – Low Carb Diet Plan

The low carb diet is a famous diet that helps you to lose weight fast because during this diet, you often limit the consumption of carbohydrates. This diet promotes the consumption of protein, fiber, and healthy fat. You have to cut the consumption of grains, starchy fruit, and vegetables that are high in carbohydrates. A low-carb diet is used to reduce weight. It helps you to reduce the risk factors linked to the metabolic syndrome and diabetes. By restricting some particular type of carbohydrates, you may be able to lose weight. It is important to change your overall eating habits. You can select lots of low-carb food items and make sure to check your doctor if you are suffering from any health condition, such as diabetes or heart disease.

Details of Diet

The low-carb diet means restriction of carbohydrates and high-calorie food items. The carbohydrates are macronutrients found in various food items and beverages. These are found in various grains, fruits, vegetables, milk, seeds, legumes, and nuts naturally. The processed food also has refined carbohydrates in the form of sugar and flour. The carbohydrates found in white bread, cookies, cake, pasta, sodas, drinks and candy are simple carbohydrates. Human body typically uses carbohydrates as a main source of fuel because the sugars and starches are broken down during the digestion process. These elements are absorbed into the bloodstream.

Fiber with carbohydrates may resist digestion and this has less effect on the blood sugar. The complex carbohydrates provide energy for your body to perform various functions. An increase in the level of sugar may trigger your body to release insulin. With the help of insulin, the glucose can easily enter in your body cells. The glucose offers energy to your body and fuel all of your activities. It is important to perform all activities from simple breathing to a jog. The additional glucose will be stored in your liver for the later use of your body. The additional glucose is converted into fat.

The low-carb diet is often followed to decrease the insulin levels and it may help your body to burn body fat for energy. It will finally lead you to lose weight.

Typical Food Items for a Low Carb Diet

Basically, the low-carb diet is focused on the protein, including fish, eggs, poultry and meat, and vegetables without starch. The use of grains, legumes, sweets, bread, starchy fruits and vegetables, nuts and seeds is strictly prohibited. You may enjoy small amounts of fruits, vegetables, and whole grains under particular circumstances. The regular limit of the carbohydrate is 60 to 130 grams and these amounts may offer you 240 to 520 calories.

Some low-carb diets require you to strictly cut the consumption of carbohydrates. While following a low-carb diet, you should restrict to 60 grams carbohydrates on a regular basis. As per dietary guidelines, the carbohydrates may be the 45 to 65 percent of your regular calorie intake. For instance, if you have to consume 2,000 calories, then you have to get 900 to 1,300 calories from carbohydrates in a day.

Weight Lose with Low-carb Diet

Some people find it difficult to reduce weight and the low-carb diets will help you to get better results. The restricted calories will help you to reduce additional body fat because the absence of carbohydrates from your diet, your body will use fat reserves. In the absence of carbohydrates, you will consume protein and fiber-rich food that may keep you full. The low-carb diet is quite better than other diets because it will help you to get lots of other advantages too. While eating protein and fiber, you can build strong muscles and reduce body fat.

Other Health Benefits of Low-Carb Diet

The low-carb diet is not only beneficial to reduce weight, but you can get the advantage of various other health benefits. It will help you to improve various health conditions, such as diabetes, high blood pressure, metabolic diseases and cardiovascular diseases. The diet will help you to improve the level of blood cholesterol and sugar level.

The low-carb diet proves helpful to improve the HDL cholesterol and the values of triglyceride. The quality of food choices and a number of carbs matters a lot in the success of your diet. You have to consume lean protein, healthy fats, and unprocessed carbohydrates.

Low Carb Food List to Eat

If you want to follow low carb diet, then it will be based on unprocessed and natural food items, such as:

•	You can enjoy beef, lamb, pork, chicken and others to increase protein and fiber consumption.

•	Without fish, the low carb diet is incomplete. The salmon, trout, haddock and many others are the best choices for you.

- You need an omega-3 supplement or pastured eggs should be consumed.

- If you want to consume vegetables, then broccoli, spinach, cauliflower, carrots and various others are good for you.

- The suitable fruits are apples, pears, oranges, blueberries, and strawberries.

- The nuts and seeds will be an important part of your diet and you can consume almonds, walnuts, seeds, sunflower, etc.

- The cheese, yogurt, butter, and heavy cream are good choices for you.

- The coconut oil, butter, olive oil, lard and cod fish liver oil are good.

Risks of Low-Carb Diet

If you drastically cut the carbohydrates from your diet, then you may experience a number health effects, such as weakness, bad breath, fatigue, headache, constipation, diarrhea, etc. There is no need to worry about these risks because these are temporary side-effects.

The long-term deficiency of the carbohydrates may result in the vitamin and mineral deficiency. You may suffer from gastrointestinal problems and bone loss. It may lead you to various chronic problems. If you want to avoid all these risks, then it is not good to cut the carbohydrates from your diet on a long-term basis.

Severe restriction of carbohydrates may result in a procedure called ketosis. It may occur in the absence of sugar because if you don't have enough sugar for energy, then your body will break down stored fat. It may lead you to ketone build up in your body. The side-effects of ketosis may include a headache, nausea, mental and physical exhaustion and bad breath.

Chapter 9 – Common Low Carb Diet Mistakes to Avoid

There are a few mistakes that should be avoided in low carb diet because these mistakes can decrease the benefits of your diet:

Consumption of Excessive Carbs

It is difficult to find out the accurate quantity of carbohydrate in food items. People often increase the consumption of carbohydrates without realizing it. You should avoid this mistake by reading the proportion of carbohydrates in a food item. People often get the advantage of a restricted range of carbohydrates and reduce weight. Make sure to avoid starchy vegetables and fruits, processed meals and other unhealthy food items.

Increase Consumption of Protein in Diet

Protein is really important macronutrient, but lots of people are not getting adequate protein. Right consumption of protein can increase the fat burning speed and this diet will lead you to reduce weight. Low-carb dieter often increases the consumption of lean meat and this can increase the consumption of protein. Extra protein can increase your weight; therefore, you should control the consumption of protein to 1.5 to 2.0 grams per kg of your body weight and 0.7 to 0.9 grams per pound. Extra protein can turn into glucose via gluconeogenesis process and extra protein consumption can avoid you from getting into ketosis.

Afraid of Fat

Some people get maximum calories from dietary carbohydrates, such as grains and sugar. Once you remove an energy source from your diet, you have to replace it with a healthy source, such as olive oil and coconut oil. Healthy fats are omega-3s, saturated, monounsaturated, and vegetable oils. Carefully include healthy fats in your diet, such as lard, butter, and coconut oil can provide 50 to 60 percent calories to your diet.

Don't Replenish Sodium

One important mechanism behind low carb diet is a reduction of insulin levels. Insulin performs various functions in the body, such as inform your fat cells to store body fat. Insulin also tells your kidneys to hold sodium. While following a low-carb diet, your insulin level may go down and body will shed extra water and sodium. This is helpful for people to get rid of extra bloat within a few days of low carb diet. Sodium is an essential electrolyte in your body this can be a problem, once your kidneys abandon excessively. You should maintain the consumption of sodium in your body. While following any diet, you have to be patient because positive results may take a longer period of time. It will be good to follow this diet for a consistent period of time.

Conclusion

If you are unable to reduce weight despite your dieting and exercise, it is time to cut off carbohydrates from your diet. The low-carb diet is designed to get rid of additional weight by reducing the consumption of wheat, white rice, and gluten. Your diet should be based on fiber, protein and gluten-free food items. Your breakfast, lunch, and dinner should be based on the gluten-free food items.

There are numerous benefits of a low-carb diet, such as you can reduce weight, avoid cardiovascular diseases and high blood pressure. It is healthy for you to try low-carb food items and get rid of lots of health complications. You can make breakfast, lunch and dinner free from carbohydrates. If you are suffering from any health complication, then it will be good to consult your doctor before following this diet.

Part 2

Introduction

The low carb diet is one of the most proven and effective diets for losing weight. The low carbohydrate diet is simple to follow, and is based on consuming foods that are mainly low in carbohydrates. Consuming less carbs in your diet, has been shown to increase the fat burned by your body, and is overall a very effective weight loss diet.

Low carb dieting tips for beginners:

- Include vegetables and lean meats (fish and chicken) in your diet. Most vegetables and meats contain low amounts of carbs, and can control your appetite.

- Avoid starchy foods like pasta, potatoes, and rice. These foods have high amounts of carbs!

- Stick to drinking water, most other drinks like juice may include sugars that you may not be aware of.

- Most processed foods have added sugars, it is recommended to avoid preserved and processed foods for this reason.

All of the recipes in this cookbook are low in carbs, high protein, and taste great. Because of how easy these recipes are to make, these low carb high protein recipes are perfect for beginners, or busy people.

We hope you enjoy these low carb high protein recipes, good luck!

Chapter 1: Low Carb High Protein Chicken Recipes

Lime Garlic Chicken

Ingredients

4 boneless, skinless chicken breast halves

2 tablespoons butter

1 tablespoon olive oil

2 teaspoons garlic powder

3 tablespoons lime juice

3/4 teaspoon salt

1/4 teaspoon black pepper

1/4 teaspoon cayenne pepper

1/8 teaspoon paprika

1/4 teaspoon garlic powder

1/8 teaspoon onion powder

1/4 teaspoon dried thyme

1/4 teaspoon dried parsley

Directions

In a small bowl, mix together salt, black pepper, cayenne, paprika, 1/4 teaspoon garlic powder, onion powder, thyme and parsley. Sprinkle spice mixture generously on both sides of chicken breasts.

Heat butter and olive oil in a large heavy skillet over medium heat. Saute chicken until golden brown, about 6 minutes on each side. Sprinkle with 2 teaspoons garlic powder and lime juice.

Cook 5 minutes more, stirring frequently to coat evenly with sauce.

Nutrition: 220 Calories; 10g Fat; 28g Protein; 2g Net Carbs per 1/4 of recipe

Creamy Chicken Bake

Ingredients

8 boneless chicken breasts, flattened

Salt, pepper and garlic powder

1/4 cup olive oil

1 pound pork sausage

1 stalk celery, chopped

8 ounces cream cheese, softened

8 ounces cheddar cheese, shredded, divided

1 pound fresh mushrooms, sliced

1/4 cup fresh parsley, chopped

Directions

Season the chicken; brown in hot oil. Set aside. Brown the sausage and celery; drain and cool slightly. Heat the oven to 350Fº.

Spray a 9x13 inch baking pan and put the mushrooms in the bottom. In a bowl, mix the sausage, cream cheese, 4 ounces cheddar cheese and the parsley.

Spoon this mixture over the mushrooms and smooth with a spoon; place the chicken on top.

Cover and bake 30 minutes. Remove the cover; top with the rest of cheese. Bake 15 minutes until the cheese is melted and browned and the chicken is fully cooked.

To serve, put the chicken on a plate cheese side up; spoon the mushroom mixture over the top.

Nutrition: 599 Calories; 43g Fat; 49g Protein; 3g Net Carbs per 1/8 of recipe

Creamy Chicken Chowder

Ingredients

3 large chicken breasts

1 package of bacon

2 cups of chicken Broth (low carb/sodium)

1 8oz package of cream cheese

2 cups of heavy cream

2 tbsp butter

1/2 large onion

1/2 bell pepper

1 stalk of celery chopped.

8 oz steams and pieces mushrooms

2 tsp minced garlic

1 tsp salt

1 tsp black pepper

1 tsp basil

1 tsp thyme

2 tsp garlic powder

Directions

Turn slow cooker on low and add vegetables and 1 1/2 cups of chicken broth in the slow cooker with butter and a pinch of Salt, cover.

Cut bacon into small pieces and cook until very crisp. Remove from pan and put aside. Leave 2 tbsp of Bacon grease in the bacon and place chicken breasts in the pan to sear on both sides.

Remove Chicken and cut into small cubes. Use remaining 1/2 cup of chicken broth to de-glaze the pan, pour this into the slow cooker.

Add bacon, chicken, heavy cream, cream cheese and seasonings, stirring until well blended.

Cook on low setting for 6 hours, stirring well before serving.

Nutrition: 382 Calories; 31g Fat; 20g Protein; 5g Net Carbs per 1/12 of recipe

Honey Mustard Chicken Breasts

Ingredients

4 boneless chicken breasts

2 tbsp Extra virgin olive oil

2 tbsp mustard

2 tbsp tarragon - dry

2 tbsp honey

Directions

Mix wet ingredients with chicken in dish or plastic bag.

Marinate chicken for up to 24 hours before cooking. Preheat oven to 350 for 20 minutes. Place chicken in glass dish or pan, using remaining marinade to put beneath chicken.

Bake chicken for approximately 30 minutes or until chicken is no longer pink.

Nutrition: 138 Calories; 5g Fat; 20g Protein; 2g Net Carbs per 1/4 of recipe

Dill Chicken Breasts

Ingredients

4 boneless, skinless chicken breast halve

1 teaspoon garlic powder

3 tablespoons butter

1/2 cup whipping cream

2 tablespoons capers, drained and rinsed

1 teaspoon lemon pepper

1 teaspoon salt

1 teaspoon dried dill weed

Directions

Season chicken breasts with lemon pepper, salt, dill weed, and garlic powder.

Melt butter in a large skillet over medium heat. Place breasts in skillet, and increase heat to medium-high.

Turn chicken frequently, until brown, about 5 minutes. Reduce heat to medium, and cook 5 to 7 minutes, until breasts are cooked through. Remove chicken to a warm serving platter, and cover with foil.

Return skillet to stove, and increase heat to high. Whisk in whipping cream, whisking continuously until reduced to sauce consistency, about 3 minutes.

Remove from heat. Stir in capers. Pour sauce over chicken, and serve.

Nutrition: 313 Calories; 21g Fat; 28g Protein; 2g Net Carbs per 1/4 of recipe

Balsamic Basil Chicken Breasts

Ingredients

6 skinless, boneless chicken breast halves

1 teaspoon garlic salt

ground black pepper to taste

2 tablespoons olive oil

1 onion, thinly sliced

1 (14.5 ounce) can diced tomatoes

1/2 cup balsamic vinegar

1 teaspoon dried basil

1 teaspoon dried oregano

1 teaspoon dried rosemary

1/2 teaspoon dried thyme

Directions

Season both sides of chicken breasts with garlic salt and pepper.

Heat olive oil in a skillet over medium heat; cook seasoned chicken breasts until chicken is browned, 3 to 4 minutes per side. Add onion; cook and stir until onion is browned, 3 to 4 minutes.

Pour diced tomatoes and balsamic vinegar over chicken; season with basil, oregano, rosemary and thyme.

Simmer until chicken is no longer pink and the juices run clear, about 15 minutes and a instant-read thermometer inserted into the center reads at least 165 F

Nutrition: 196 Calories; 7g Fat; 24g Protein; 7g Net Carbs per 1/6 of recipe

Mediterranean Chicken Breasts

Ingredients

6 skinless, boneless chicken breast halves

6 ounces tomato basil feta cheese, crumbled

1/4 cup Italian-style dry bread crumbs, divided

Directions

Preheat oven to 350 F. Lightly grease a 9x13 inch baking dish.

Place chicken breasts between 2 pieces of waxed paper. Gently pound chicken with flat side of meat mallet until approximately 1/4 inch thick; remove wax paper. Place 1 ounce of feta cheese in the center of each chicken breast, and fold in half.

Spread 2 tablespoons bread crumbs in the bottom of the prepared baking dish. Arrange chicken in the dish, and top with remaining bread crumbs.

Bake 30 minutes in the preheated oven, or until chicken is no longer pink and juices run clear.

Nutrition: 224 Calories; 8g Fat; 32g Protein; 4.5g Net Carbs per 1/6 of recipe

Marinara Chicken

Ingredients

2 pounds boneless, skinless chicken breasts

4 cloves garlic, peeled and crushed

4 tomatoes, chopped or one 14.5-ounce can low-sodium tomatoes, drained

4 medium ribs celery, diced

2 small zucchini, diced

1 bell pepper, cored, seeded, and diced

One 18-oz jar low-sodium marinara sauce

1 tsp dried basil

1 tsp dried thyme

Directions

Place the chicken in the slow cooker; add the garlic, tomatoes, celery, zucchini, and pepper.

Pour the marinara sauce over all, and sprinkle the basil and thyme on top.

Set the slow cooker on low and cook for 6 to 7 hours. Before serving, shred the chicken with a fork.

Nutrition: 178 Calories; 4g Fat; 27g Protein; 8g Net Carbs per 1/8 of recipe

Chicken Creole

Ingredients

8-12 chicken thighs, skin removed

1 cup celery, chopped, 4 ounces

1 red pepper, sliced, 4 ounces

1 green pepper, sliced, 4 ounces

Small onion, chopped, 2 1/2 ounces

4 ounce can mushrooms, drained

14.5 ounce can diced tomatoes

1 teaspoon garlic powder

1 teaspoon granular Splenda or equivalent liquid Splenda

1 teaspoon Cajun Seasoning

1/2 teaspoon paprika

1 teaspoon salt

1/2 teaspoon pepper

Hot sauce, to taste

Directions

Put the chicken in a crockpot. Mix the remaining ingredients and pour over the chicken. Cook on low 7-8 hours.

Nutrition: 325 Calories; 22g Fat; 26g Protein; 4g Net Carbs per 1/8 of recipe

Spicy Grilled Chicken Breasts

Ingredients

3 chicken breasts

1 tsp salt

2 garlic cloves

1 tbsp ginger

1/2 onion chopped

1 jalapeno pepper, minced

3/4 cup unsweetened coconut milk

1 cup frozen peas

Directions

Heat a non-stick frying pan, cut chicken in thirds and then add chicken to skillet. Let chicken cook without moving it for 3 minutes, to let the chicken brown.

Flip over and add the garlic, ginger, onion and jalapeno. Stir and cook until onion is started to get soft.

Add the coconut milk and stir. Cook on lower heat for another 7-10 minutes.

Toss in the peas and cook for another two minutes until the chicken is fully cooked and no longer pink.

Nutrition: 320 Calories; 11g Fat; 44g Protein; 9g Net Carbs per 1/4 of recipe

Chicken And Swiss Cheese Casserole

Ingredients

1 pound boneless chicken breasts or tenders, cut into bite-size pieces

12 ounces ham, cut into cubes

6 ounces Swiss cheese, shredded

Salt and pepper, to taste

8 ounces cream cheese, softened

1/2 cup heavy cream

1 clove garlic, minced

1/8 teaspoon freshly ground pepper

1/8 teaspoon dill

2 teaspoons chives

1 tablespoon fresh parsley, chopped

Directions

Put the chicken, ham and cheese in a greased 12x7 inch baking dish. Season with a little salt and pepper.

In a medium bowl, blend the heavy cream into the cream cheese until smooth. Stir in the garlic, pepper, dill, chives and parsley. Pour over the meat and cheese and stir everything together.

Bake at 350F° for about 40 minutes until bubbly and the chicken is fully cooked.

Let stand about 10 minutes before serving to allow some of the liquid to soak back into the sauce.

Nutrition: 754 Calories; 55g Fat; 60g Protein; 4g Net Carbs per 1/4 of recipe

BBQ Chicken Wings

Ingredients

3 pounds chicken wings (15 wings)

Salt and freshly ground black pepper

½ cup hickory flavored barbecue sauce

1-1/2 tablespoons dijon mustard

1 tablespoon red wine vinegar

1 tablespoon honey

1 tablespoon hot sauce

Directions

Preheat oven to 400 degrees. Cut off and discard wing tips. Cut each wing at joint to make two sections.

Place wing pieces on foil lined baking sheet. Season to taste with salt and pepper. Bake for about 20 minutes or until chicken is a light, golden brown.

Transfer chicken wings to slow cooker. In a bowl, whisk together the barbecue sauce, mustard, vinegar, honey and hot sauce.

Pour over the chicken wing pieces and toss gently until completely coated.

Cover and cook on LOW for 4 to 4-1/2 hours or until the wings are tender.

Stir at least once to make sure that the wings are evenly coated with the sauce.

Nutrition: 331 Calories; 22g Fat; 7g Carbohydrates; 24g Protein; per 1/8 of recipe

Chapter 2: High Protein Low Carb Beef Recipes

Black Pepper And Garlic Flank Steak

Ingredients

1 (2 pound) flank steak or round steak

3 cloves garlic, minced

1/2 cup soy sauce

2 tablespoons vegetable oil

2 tablespoons ketchup

1 teaspoon dried oregano

1 teaspoon ground black pepper

3 cloves garlic, minced

1/2 cup soy sauce

2 tablespoons vegetable oil

2 tablespoons ketchup

1 teaspoon dried oregano

1 teaspoon ground black pepper

Directions

In a small bowl, mix together garlic, soy sauce, oil, ketchup, oregano, and black pepper. Pierce meat with a fork on both sides.

Place meat and marinade in a large resealable plastic bag. Refrigerate 8 hours, or overnight.

Preheat grill for medium-high heat.

Lightly oil the grill grate. Place steak on the grill, and discard marinade.

Cook for 5 to 8 minutes per side, depending on thickness. Do not overcook, as it is better on the rare side.

Nutrition: 222 Calories; 9g Fat; 4g Carbohydrates; 30g Protein; per 1/6 of recipe

Adobo Chipotle Steak

Ingredients

4 (8 ounce) beef sirloin steaks

1 lime, juiced

1 tablespoon minced garlic

1 teaspoon dried oregano

1 teaspoon ground cumin

2 tablespoons finely chopped canned chipotle peppers in adobo sauce

adobo sauce from canned chipotle peppers to taste

salt and pepper to taste

Directions

In a small bowl, mix the lime juice, garlic, oregano, and cumin. Stir in chipotle peppers, and season to taste with adobo sauce.

Pierce the meat on both sides with a sharp knife, sprinkle with salt and pepper, and place in a glass dish. Pour lime and chipotle sauce over meat, and turn to coat. Cover, and marinate in the refrigerator for 1 to 2 hours.

Preheat grill for high heat.

Lightly brush grill grate with oil. Place steaks on the grill, and discard marinade.

Grill steaks for 6 minutes per side, or to desired doneness.

Nutrition: 342 Calories; 18g Fat; 4g Carbohydrates; 38g Protein; per 1/4 of recipe

Beef Stir Fry

Ingredients

8 oz top sirloin beef

3 cloves garlic

2 tsp soy sauce

1/2 of a leek

Dash of salt and pepper

Directions

Slice beef and combine with garlic, soy sauce, and pepper and marinate at room temperature for 20 minutes.

Slice leeks and set aside.

In a skillet, heat oil over high heat and begin to brown the beef. Add leeks and salt and stir until leeks are wilted and meat cooked.

Nutrition: 151 Calories; 5g Fat; 3g Carbohydrates; 21g Protein; per 1/4 of recipe

Spicy Jalapeno Sirloin

Ingredients

1 1/2 pounds top sirloin steak

4 jalapeno peppers, stemmed

4 cloves garlic, peeled

1 1/2 teaspoons cracked black pepper

1 tablespoon coarse salt

1/4 cup lime juice

1 tablespoon dried oregano

Directions

Combine jalapenos, garlic, pepper, salt, lime juice and oregano in a blender. Blend until smooth.

Place steak in a shallow pan or large resealable plastic bag. Pour jalapeno marinade over the steak, and turn to coat. Cover pan or seal bag; marinate in the refrigerator 8 hours or overnight.

Preheat an outdoor grill for high heat, and lightly oil the grill grate.

Drain and discard marinade. Grill steak 5 minutes per side, or to desired doneness.

Nutrition: 186 Calories; 10g Fat; 3g Carbohydrates; 19g Protein; per 1/4 of recipe

BBQ Short Ribs

Ingredients

4 pounds boneless beef short ribs

13 ounces low carb barbecue sauce

Directions

Place the ribs in a crock pot and pour in the barbecue sauce. Cook on LOW about 8 hours until the meat is tender.

Nutrition: 779 Calories; 58g Fat; 55g Protein; 6g Net Carbs per 1/6 of recipe

Marinated Ginger Steak

Ingredients

4 (8 ounce) beef sirloin steaks, at least 3/4 inch thick

2 tablespoons soy sauce

1 teaspoon ground ginger

1/2 teaspoon salt

1 teaspoon ground black pepper

1 teaspoon dried basil

1 tablespoon prepared yellow mustard

1 teaspoon lemon juice

Directions

Preheat the ovens broiler.

In a small bowl, mix together the soy sauce, ginger, salt, pepper, basil, mustard and lemon juice until smooth. Place the steaks on a broiling pan, and pour 1/4 of the mixture over each one. Rub into the meat.

Broil the steaks for 5 minutes, then turn over and cook to your desired level of doneness.

Nutrition: 296 Calories; 13g Fat; 2g Carbohydrates; 40g Protein; per 1/4 of recipe

Garlic And Herb Beef Tenderloin

Ingredients

5 pound whole beef tenderloin

6 tablespoons olive oil

8 large garlic cloves, minced

2 tablespoons minced fresh rosemary

1 tablespoon dried thyme leaves

2 tablespoons coarsely ground black pepper

1 tablespoon salt

Directions

Prepare beef: Trim off excess fat with a sharp knife. Fold thin tip end under to approximate the thickness of the rest of the roast. Tie with butcher's twine, then keep tying the roast with twine every 11/2 to 2 inches.

Cut silverskin with scissors to keep roast from bowing during cooking. Then, mix oil, garlic, rosemary, thyme, pepper and salt; rub over roast to coat. Set meat aside.

Either build a charcoal fire in half the grill or turn all gas burners on high for 10 minutes. Lubricate grate with an oil-soaked rag using tongs.

Place beef on hot rack and close lid; grill until well-seared, about 5 minutes. Turn meat and close lid; grill until well-seared on second side, another 5 minutes.

Move meat to the charcoal grills cool side, or turn off burner directly underneath the meat and turn remaining one or two burners to medium.

Cook until a meat thermometer inserted in the thickest section registers 130 degrees for rosy pink, 45 to 60 minutes, depending on tenderloin size and grill.

Let meat rest 15 minutes before carving.

Nutrition: 346 Calories; 27g Fat; 2g Carbohydrates; 26g Protein; per 1/13 of recipe

Blue Cheese Peppercorn Steak

Ingredients

1 beef fillet (12 ounces), cut into 3-ounce steaks

3 tbsp crumbled blue cheese

1/4 cup chopped parsley

2 tsp of black, red, and pink peppercorns

Directions

Preheat the oven to 375° F.

In a small bowl, combine the blue cheese and parsley and use a wooden spoon to loosely work into a paste. Cover and refrigerate.

Spread the cracked peppercorns onto a plate. Pat the meat dry and roll in the peppercorns to coat on all sides.

Place a cast-iron skillet or heavy-bottomed ovenproof sauté pan over moderately high heat.

Once hot, place steaks into the dry pan and sear the top and bottom of each steak, 1 to 2 minutes per side.

Place 1 tablespoon of the blue cheese mixture on top of each steak and transfer the pan to the oven. Roast 6 to 7 minutes for rare, 7 to 8 minutes for medium.

Nutrition: 245 Calories; 18g Fat; 1g Carbohydrates; 19g Protein; per 1/4 of recipe

Spiced Roasted Beef Tenderloin

Ingredients

2 (2 pound) beef tenderloin roasts, trimmed

2 tablespoons fresh rosemary

2 tablespoons fresh thyme leaves

2 bay leaves

4 cloves garlic

1 large shallot, peeled and quartered

1 tablespoon grated orange zest

1 tablespoon coarse salt

1 teaspoon freshly ground black pepper

1/2 teaspoon ground nutmeg

1/4 teaspoon ground cloves

2 tablespoons olive oil

Directions

In a food processor, combine rosemary, thyme, bay leaves, garlic, shallot, orange zest, salt, pepper, nutmeg, and cloves. Run machine while adding oil; process until smooth.

Spread mixture evenly over all sides of tenderloins. Place beef in a large glass baking dish. Cover with foil, and refrigerate for at least 6 hours.

Preheat oven to 400F.

Place tenderloins on a rack in a large roasting pan. Roast beef in preheated oven until meat thermometer registers 140 degrees when inserted into center of beef, about 35 minutes.

Remove from oven, and cover loosely with foil; let stand for 10 minutes. Slice beef, and serve.

Nutrition: 683 Calories; 55g Fat; 2g Carbohydrates; 41g Protein; per 1/8 of recipe

Spicy Shredded Beef With Salsa

Ingredients

3 lb beef chuck roast, trim fat

1 tbsp cumin seed

1 tbsp coriander seed

1 tbsp chili powder

1 tsp salt

1 tbsp cayenne pepper

1 cup salsa

2 tbsp water

1 tbsp cornstarch

Directions

Cut roast in half. Combine cumin, coriander, chili powder, salt and red pepper in small bowl.

Rub over roast. Place 1/4 cup salsa in slow cooker; top with one piece roast. Layer 1/4 cup salsa, remaining beef and 1/2 cup salsa in slow cooker. Cover; cook on LOW 8 to 10 hours.

Remove roast from cooking liquid; cool slightly. Trim and discard excess fat from beef. Shred meat with forks.

Let cooking liquid stand 5 minute. Skim off fat. Blend water and cornstarch until smooth.

Whisk into liquid in slow cooker. Cook, uncovered, 15 minutes on HIGH until thickened. Return beef to slow cooker.

Cover; cook 15 minutes or until hot. Adjust seasonings.

Nutrition: 324 Calories; 15g Fat; 44g Protein; 2g Net Carbs per 1/16 of recipe

Beef Tenderloin With Herbs

Ingredients

1 (3 pound) beef tenderloin

2 teaspoons olive oil

2 cloves garlic, minced

2 teaspoons dried basil

1 1/2 teaspoons dried rosemary, crushed

1 teaspoon sea salt

fresh ground black pepper to taste

Directions

Preheat oven to 425 F.

Tie the tenderloin at 2-inch intervals with kitchen string.

Combine oil and garlic in a bowl; brush over meat. Mix basil, rosemary, sea salt, and black pepper together in a bowl; sprinkle evenly over the meat.

Roast beef tenderloin in preheated oven until beginning to firm and is hot and slightly pink in the center, 40 to 50 minutes.

An instant-read thermometer inserted into the center should read 140 degrees F.

Nutrition: 205 Calories; 14g Fat; 1g Carbohydrates; 17g Protein; per 1/12 of recipe

Chapter 3: Low Carb High Protein Pork Recipes

Balsamic Pork Tenderloin With Glaze

Ingredients

1 1/2 lb pork tenderloin

1/4 tsp salt

1/8 tsp black pepper

1/4 cup balsamic vinegar

3 tbsp Splenda brown sugar blend

Directions

Preheat oven to 425F.

Rinse pork and pat dry season with salt and pepper, then brown pork in a skillet until all sides are caramelized. Turn heat to medium low and remove pork from pan.

Add the balsamic vinegar to skillet, stir and loosen up all the brown crusty material from bottom of pan, add the Splenda. Continue to stir until it is fully mixed and forms a glaze, then place pork back in pan turning to coat.

Place pan in roasting pan and place in oven roast for 25 minutes or until pork is cooked. Glaze pork periodically with the remaining glaze in the pan.

Nutrition: 257 Calories; 9g Fat; 7g Carbohydrates; 33g Protein; per 1/6 of recipe

Southwest Pork Tenderloin

Ingredients

2 whole pork tenderloins

4 teaspoons chili powder

1 1/2 teaspoons dried oregano

3/4 teaspoon ground cumin

1/8 teaspoon dried garlic powder

Directions

Mix together chili powder, oregano, cumin, and garlic powder. Rub over the surface of pork. Cover and refrigerate 2-24 hours.

Grill over medium hot coals or broil in oven turning occasionally. Cook for 20-25 minutes until meat is fully cooked. Meat thermometer should read 155-160° F when placed in center.

Nutrition: 170 Calories; 5g Fat; 1g Carbohydrates; 28g Protein; per 1/6 of recipe

Marinated Ginger Pork Chops

Ingredients

6 pork loin chops, 1/2 inch thick

1/2 cup orange juice

2 tablespoons soy sauce

2 tablespoons minced fresh ginger root

2 tablespoons grated orange zest

1 teaspoon minced garlic

1 teaspoon garlic chile paste

1/2 teaspoon salt

Directions

In a shallow container, mix together orange juice, soy sauce, ginger, orange zest, garlic, chile paste, and salt. Add pork chops, and turn to coat evenly. Cover, and refrigerate for at least 2 hours, or overnight. Turn the pork chops in the marinade occasionally.

Preheat grill for high heat, and lightly oil grate.

Grill pork chops for 5 to 6 minutes per side, or to desired doneness.

Nutrition: 136 Calories; 3g Fat; 4g Carbohydrates; 21g Protein; per 1/6 of recipe

Green Chili Pork

Ingredients

2 tbsp ground cumin

1 tsp cayenne pepper

1 tbsp salt

1 tbsp chile powder

1 boneless pork roast (3 lbs)

3 (4 oz each) cans diced green chiles

Juice of 2 limes

9 cloves garlic, crushed

1 cup low-fat, low-sodium chicken broth

1 medium onion, diced

1 tbsp minced fresh cilantro

Directions

Combine spices and rub over pork.

Place pork into slow cooker. Combine remaining ingredients and pour over meat.

Cook on low for 7-10 hours. Remove meat from slow cooker and lightly shred with a fork.

Place back into slow cooker and stir. Drain juice from meat and serve.

Nutrition: 278 Calories; 16g Fat; 28g Protein; 5g Net Carbs per 1/10 of recipe

Pork Loin Roast With Herbs

Ingredients

1 (4-pound) boneless pork loin, with fat left on

1 tablespoon salt

2 tablespoons olive oil

4 cloves garlic, minced

1 teaspoon dried thyme or 2 teaspoons minced fresh thyme leaves

1 teaspoon dried basil or 2 teaspoons fresh basil leaves

1 teaspoon dried rosemary or 2 teaspoons minced fresh rosemary

Directions

Preheat oven to 475 degrees F.

Place the pork loin on a rack in a roasting pan. Combine the remaining ingredients in a small bowl. With your fingers, massage the mixture onto the pork loin, covering all of the meat and fat.

Roast the pork for 30 minutes, then reduce the heat to 425 degrees F and roast for an additional hour.

Test for doneness using an instant-read thermometer. When the internal temperature reaches 155 degrees F, remove the roast from the oven.

Allow it to sit for about 20 minutes before carving.

Nutrition: 209 Calories; 10g Fat; 1g Carbohydrates; 27g Protein; per 1/6 of recipe

Garlic Pork Chops

Ingredients

4 thick cut boneless pork chops

1/4 cup olive oil

1 cup chicken broth

2 cloves garlic, minced

1 tablespoon paprika

1 tablespoon garlic powder

1 tablespoon poultry seasoning

1 teaspoon dried oregano

1 teaspoon dried basil

salt and pepper to taste

Directions

In a large bowl, whisk together the olive oil, chicken broth, garlic, paprika, garlic powder, poultry seasoning, oregano, and basil. Pour into the slow cooker.

Cut small slits in each pork chop with the tip of a knife, and season lightly with salt and pepper.

Place pork chops into the slow cooker, cover, and cook on High for 4 hours. Baste periodically with the sauce.

Nutrition: 275 Calories; 20g Fat; 20g Protein; 4g Net Carbs per 1/4 of recipe

Herb And Lemon Pork Chops

Ingredients

6 (4 ounce) boneless pork loin chops

1/4 cup lemon juice

2 tablespoons vegetable oil

4 cloves garlic, minced

1 teaspoon salt

1/4 teaspoon dried oregano

1/4 teaspoon pepper

Directions

In a large resealable bag, combine lemon juice, oil, garlic, salt, oregano, and pepper. Place chops in bag, seal, and refrigerate 2 hours or overnight. Turn bag frequently to distribute marinade.

Preheat an outdoor grill for high heat. Remove chops from bag, and transfer remaining marinade to a saucepan. Bring marinade to a boil, remove from heat, and set aside.

Lightly oil the grill grate. Grill pork chops for 5 to 7 minutes per side, basting frequently with boiled marinade, until done.

Nutrition: 202 Calories; 10g Fat; 25g Protein; 2g Net Carbs per 1/6 of recipe

Spicy Pulled Pork

Ingredients

2.5 lb pork roast

1 can tomatoes with diced green chiles

1 small can diced green chiles

2 tsp taco seasoning

1 tsp cayenne pepper or to taste

3 cloves of garlic; minced

1/2 cup chopped onion

Directions

Place 1 can of tomatoes with diced green chiles on the bottom of slow cooker. Place pork roast on top.

Mix can of green chiles with the other ingredients and pour on top of the roast.

Set slow cooker on low for 8 hours. Once finished cooking, shred pork and place it back in the slow cooker to mix with the juices.

Nutrition: 250 Calories; 18g Fat; 18g Protein; 2g Net Carbs per 1/12 of recipe

Conclusion

It is my sincere hope that you might have liked all the recipes which have been mentioned in the book and once again thank you for getting this book and experimenting with the recipes.

About The Author

Richard Leonard is born with the vision to promote the art of *Low Carb* cooking among the masses. The author has written several research papers on the topic. He has served as an instructor promoting various cultural arts in University of San Francisco. He is currently living with his spouse in Texas.